GIVE YOURSELF PERMISSION TO BE HAPPY

DR. HOWARD MURAD, M.D.

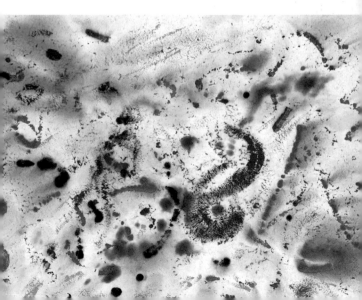

Copyright © 2014 by Howard Murad

All rights reserved. No part of this publication may be reproduced, distributed, or transmitted in any form or by any means, including photocopying, recording, or other electronic or mechanical methods, without the prior written permission of the publisher, except in the case of brief quotations embodied in critical reviews and certain other noncommercial uses permitted by copyright law. For permission requests, write to the publisher, addressed "Attention: Permissions Coordinator," at the address below.

Wisdom Waters Press
1000 Wilshire Blvd., #1500
Los Angeles, CA 90017-2457

Quantity sales. Special discounts are available on quantity purchases by corporations, associations, and others. For details, contact the "Special Sales Department" at the address above.

Printed in China

ISBN-10: 1939642213
ISBN-13: 978-1939642219

First Edition

17 16 15 14 13   10 9 8 7 6 5 4 3 2 1

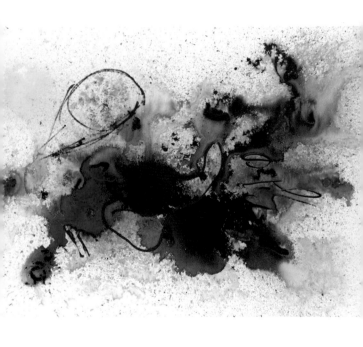

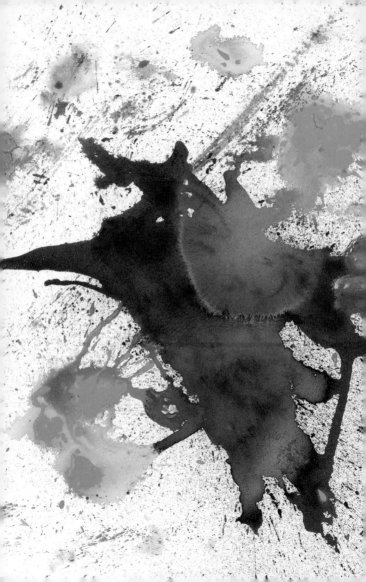

Permission is a very powerful word, one that can set you free to pursue your dreams. But don't wait for someone else to say, "I give you permission." You can give *yourself* permission to be happy, healthy, and successful!

ABOUT
THE ART

Self-expression is essential to human health and happiness. The author was reminded of that several years ago when he discovered a new outlet for his own irrepressible creative drive: painting. Interestingly enough, he's never taken any formal art classes, but his canvases are nonetheless sophisticated. His modernist style makes pure chance a key element in the artistic process. This results in explosions of color and form that expand the limits of imagination. Dr. Murad created the illustrations for this book hoping they would help you expand your imagination and envision a better tomorrow.

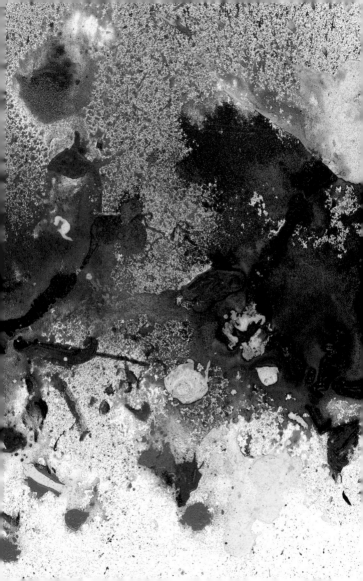

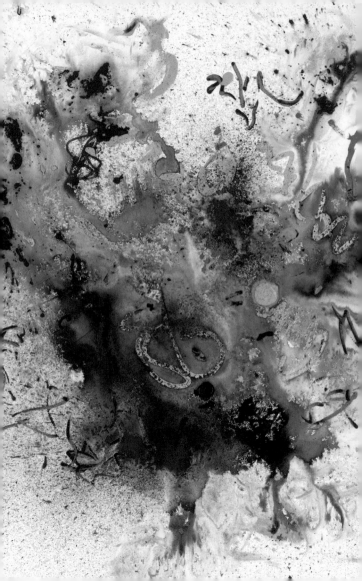

GIVE YOURSELF PERMISSION TO BE HAPPY

Over the years, I've treated more than 50,000 patients, and they have been the source of countless fascinating stories. Among my favorites is the story of a very nice young lady—let's call her Jeannie— who came to me with a recurring rash. I successfully treated the rash, but it soon became apparent that the challenges she faced were more than just skin deep.

Jeannie had a host of health concerns as well as issues in her personal and professional life. It was easy to see that she was not a very healthy or happy person. It seemed to me that all of this might be linked in some way, so I told her what I'd observed and asked an obvious question. *Why was she so unhappy?*

"I don't know," Jeannie replied. "I'm not sure I deserve to be happy. The fact is, I'm not living up to anyone's expectations, least of all my own."

"Do expectations really matter, especially the expectations of other people?" I asked. "It sounds almost as if you're waiting for someone to give you permission to be happy."

It's amazing how often I've had conversations like this one with patients, friends, family members, business associates, even other doctors. They *want* to be happy. They *want* to feel accomplished, successful, and fulfilled, but there is always something holding them back. In nearly every case, the obstacle is the same: They don't give themselves *permission*.

Permission is a very powerful word—one that can limit you for a lifetime or set you free to pursue your dreams. Do you have permission to live your life the way you want to live it? Or don't you? Actually, it's entirely up to you. Only you can give yourself permission to take risks, try new things, meet interesting people, or give up on old ways of thinking that are holding you back. You—only you—can give yourself permission to be more powerful, creative, healthy, or, most important of all, *happy.*

All too often we limit ourselves and tell ourselves that we aren't good enough to get what we want out of life. I've had friends who wanted to be doctors but who never gave themselves permission to try. Perhaps they thought they were incapable or unworthy in some way. They never applied to medical school. If they had applied, they might have failed, but it seems far more likely that they would have found the energy and strength they needed to succeed and become excellent doctors. What a big difference a little permission can make.

I think giving yourself permission allows you to take full advantage of your capabilities, which are almost certainly greater than you think. Giving yourself permission can enable you to reach your full potential. But for whatever reason, too many of us never give ourselves permission to take those crucial first steps toward a richer, more abundant life. Too many of us never give ourselves permission to try out a new career, get out of a relationship that's just not working, give up on a dead-end job or an uncomfortable house or

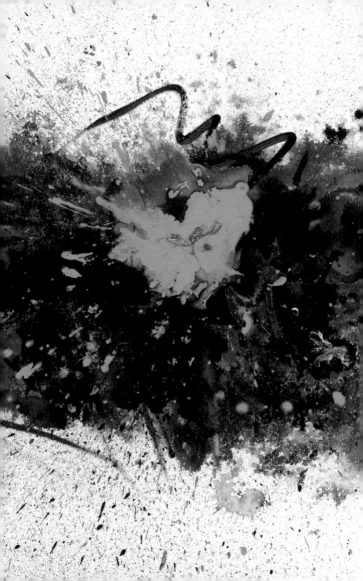

apartment, move to a more pleasant part of the country, or even to stop eating too much or too little.

I'm sure you can think of many such healthy and appropriate behavioral changes that you could make, but you don't make them because you haven't given yourself permission. Sometimes there is something in your history that has led you to withhold permission. For my patient Jeannie, her troubles could be traced to her childhood and her relationship with her mother who put tremendous emphasis on physical appearance.

"A girl should be pretty," her mother said, but Jeannie never felt she was pretty *enough*. This gave her low self-esteem and caused her to limit herself in a whole variety of ways. Since she felt unworthy, she could never give herself permission to reach for what she really wanted out of life.

Occasionally, I have what seems to me an important insight into the human quest for health and happiness. Usually these insights occur to me when I'm working with a patient or talking with a friend, and over the years I've collected hundreds of what I often describe simply as "sayings." *Give yourself permission to be happy* is one of them.

When patients visit my office or take part in our Inclusive Health program, I share several of the sayings with them. If any of the sayings seem especially meaningful to them, I make a copy and give it to them. As it turned out, the saying Jeannie focused on wasn't *Give yourself permission to be happy.* Instead, it was *Give yourself permission to be successful.*

At the time Jeannie was taking part in our Inclusive Health program she had a job

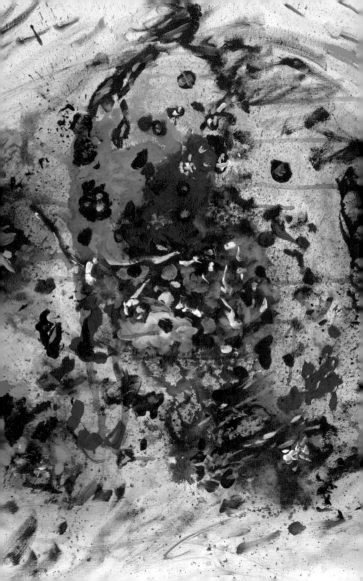

working for a big company helping executives deal with customers, employees, and the press. She was very good at teaching others to be better communicators, but she'd never tried to employ those skills herself. She lacked the self-confidence to stand up in front of people and share her ideas and passions. She had not given herself *permission* to take center stage. But that was about the change.

Inspired by the idea that she could give herself permission to succeed, her life took off in an entirely new and far more rewarding direction. She tried and tried again and eventually became a very dynamic public speaker. Before long she had quit working for others and was running her own company. Today she travels all over the world speaking to large groups about ways to improve communication skills.

Along with Jeannie's professional achievements came many other benefits. She had not just given herself permission to become successful but also to eat better, to get more exercise, to take better care of her skin, to be more positive in her relationships with others, and to live life as she really wanted to live it. Her health and her personal life had undergone a transformation right along with her career. She began to enjoy a richer and more fulfilling existence. In short, she became, and remains to this day, a happy woman.

Neither Jeannie's problems nor her solution to them are unique. If you think carefully about your own life, you'll certainly remember times when you have denied yourself permission. So ask yourself this question: Why shouldn't you give yourself permission to be the happiest and most successful person you are capable of being?

If you are not living life as you imagine it should be lived, perhaps you could benefit from following Jeannie's example. Give yourself permission to take risks, try new things, meet interesting new people, or give up on old ways of thinking that just aren't helpful anymore—and maybe never were. Give yourself a chance, and I'll bet you will make your own luck—and happiness.

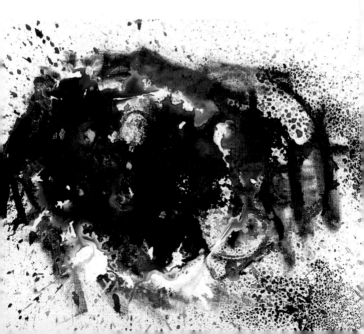

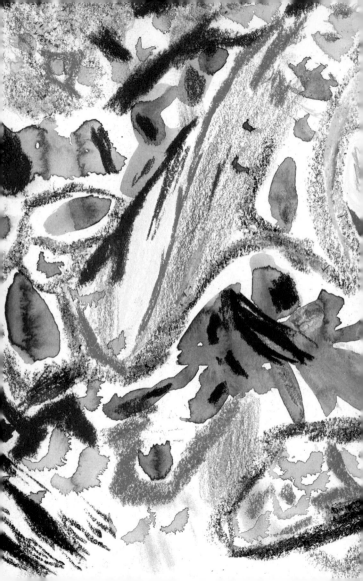

LIFE IS ART

When I create paintings like the ones you see in this book, I make a few marks on a canvas, add some colors, and spray them with water. The water is allowed to inter-act with the art in a more or less random way, and this often carries the artwork in a totally unexpected direction. How's it going to turn out? I don't know.

My life has been like that, too. I started out thinking I wanted to be an engineer. When that didn't work out for me, I went into pharmacy and that, in turn, led me into medicine. Whatever happened along the way, I always felt life was carrying me somewhere. Life is a canvas, you see. You make your mark on it and then flow with it. If you allow it to flow in a way that makes sense, your life will be a work of art.

Interestingly, I didn't start painting until 2008 when retinal surgery forced me to spend a rather challenging month always looking down. My wife, Loralee, suggested I try my hand at art to help me pass the time. I followed her advice and found that expressing myself with color on canvas was far more invigorating than I had ever imagined. I truly believe the painting helped me heal faster, and after that experience, I began to incorporate art into my overall philosophy for skincare and general health. Along with an emphasis on personal creativity, my approach includes appropriate skincare products, targeted supplements, rest, exercise, and above all, a diet featuring a wide variety of wholesome, water-rich foods.

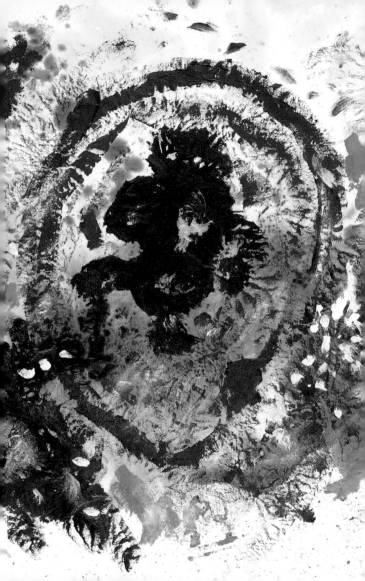

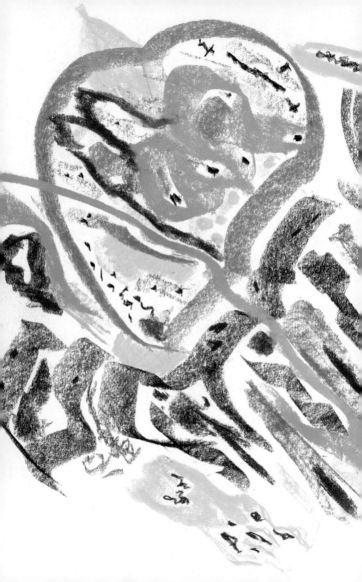

It also includes a positive attitude. If you smile a lot and turn a happy face toward other people, you're going to look a lot more attractive. There is an emotional component to both your appearance and your health, and when you are creative your emotions are allowed to run free. If you have an engaging outlet for your natural creativity, you will sleep better, be more vibrant, and smile a lot more.

When I consult with patients, we don't just talk about individual skin conditions. These are always linked to other problems and concerns, so we discuss a whole range of health-related issues. We also discuss various ways people can express themselves creatively. This will improve their overall well-being, and I try to send them home with a plan that takes personal creativity into consideration.

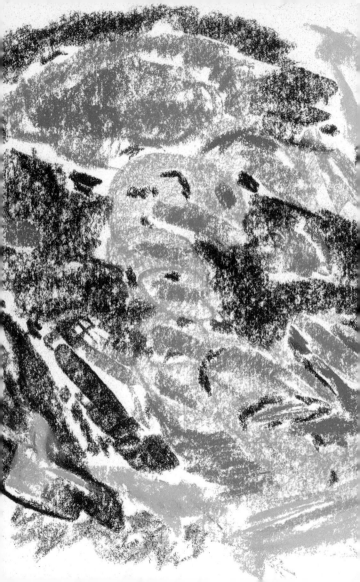

SIMPLE WORDS
OF WISDOM

Many of the sayings I share with patients are related in one way or another. They all have in common the idea that you can change your life for the better, that it's all a matter of how you approach the challenges of living and that you don't need permission from any higher authority to find happiness. Here are a few sayings that, in my way of thinking at least, are closely linked to the ones that made such a difference to Jeannie.

You are worthy
A strong sense of personal worthiness is the key to health, happiness, and success.

27

Unless you feel worthy of success, you won't experience it. Unless you feel worthy of love, you are unlikely to receive it. You *are* worthy and you should remind yourself of that constantly. Look in the mirror and say, "I am worthy. I can succeed. I can make a difference. I can change myself and the world for the better."

Give yourself permission to say no

No is a very potent word, and it is okay to say it occasionally. In fact, the right to say no is what makes us sovereign individuals. You don't always have to do what other people say. You can say no and *make up your own mind* about what you're going to do. Then you can move forward without regrets or apologies.

Don't measure yourself against unattainable goals

You'll never run a two-minute mile, you'll never swim the width of the Pacific, and you'll probably never be the richest person in the world. It's very unhelpful and unhealthful to measure yourself against goals that are either unattainable or out of the realm of possibility. It's usually best not to measure yourself against the achievements of others. Instead, set reasonable goals of your own and measure yourself against those.

Be comfortable with yourself so you can become comfortable with others

Look at yourself in the mirror. Do you like the person you see there? If you do, and if you feel comfortable with that person, then you are more likely to be comfortable with others. You are also more likely to project a positive, self-confident image and to be happy and successful. Be your own best friend. If you enjoy your own company, then you'll find it much easier to make friends and have fun with others.

Be brave enough
to make difficult decisions

Because decisions involve choices that may turn out to have been either right or wrong, decisions can be very difficult. Sometimes we avoid decisions because we're afraid of making the wrong one. But making no decision at all can be even worse! Decisions have to be made all the time, and avoiding them will paralyze you and bring any project you pursue to a grinding halt. Decision making takes guts, but you'll never make the right decision unless you're brave enough to take a chance and risk getting it wrong. To succeed, you must have the courage to fail.

Expose your accomplishments
without fear of rejection

Most of us were brought up to believe that modesty is a virtue. That may or may not be so, but too much modesty can make us

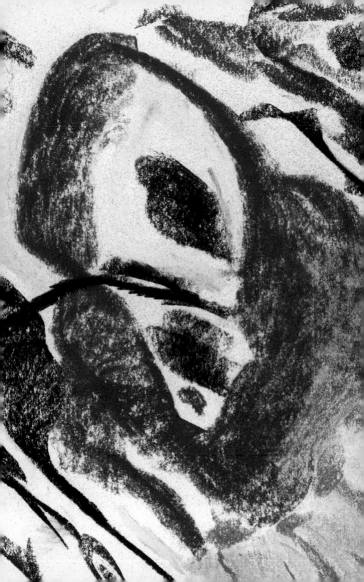

afraid to share our ideas and achievements with others. Don't be afraid they'll think you immodest or believe your accomplishments fall far short of their own. More likely, they won't think either of those things, and if they do, that's their problem, not yours. Don't worry, there will always be intellectually and emotionally generous people out there who will recognize your talents and who are prepared to celebrate your victories with you.

Allow happiness to enter

Most people experience very little happiness in their lives because they just don't open up and let it come through the door. Perhaps they believe they're unworthy or they're waiting for someone to tell them that it's okay to be happy. Happiness does not require a permit, and you don't need anyone's permission. Give yourself permission to be happy, and happiness will come knocking. There is a tremendous amount of beauty and happiness out there in the world. Invite it into your life.

Become free to be yourself

Trying to copy others won't help you become the person you were meant to be. What's wrong with being that genuine and capable person you really are? You have something unique to contribute; celebrate what you have to offer. Set yourself free, and you'll be amazed by what you can accomplish.

Free those you love

If you love someone, then you must avoid building walls around them. Instead, open doors for them and encourage them to become themselves and to do the things that bring them joy. In some wedding ceremonies, the young couple is encouraged to "grow apart together." That's a wonderful formula for a deep and loving long-term relationship.

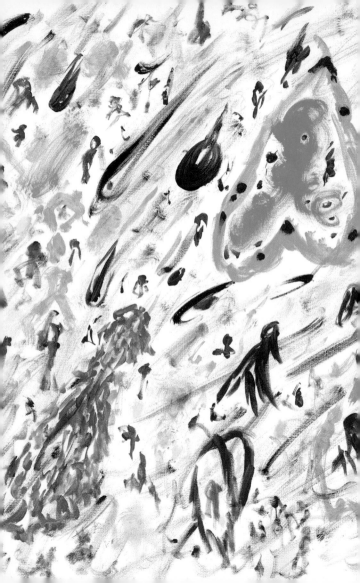

Competency trumps genius

You may think you lack the talent to succeed in sports, academics, or business, but if so, you are probably wrong. With hard work and perseverance, you can compete with anyone, even with those who at first may seem more capable. Competence often succeeds where genius, for one reason or another, may fail. You don't have to be a genius in order to succeed or to accomplish great things.

Your best is better than the competition

Always keep in mind that when you do your very best, that is likely to make you a winner. You can do better than your competitors even if they have more overall ability. Also it's important to concentrate on those talents and abilities that are the very best you have to offer. There is always something you are better at than anyone else.

Ignore the naysayers and allow yourself to achieve your maximum potential

Other people may say you won't succeed, but don't listen to them! You should also ignore the even more powerful naysayers within—those internal voices that insist you're sure to fail. Instead, give yourself positive messages—you are good enough, you will succeed, and you will accomplish your goals. To realize your true potential, free yourself from negativity. Professional athletes and other successful people always try to emphasize the positive. Follow their example and you'll have more confidence and greater success in everything you attempt.

Project self-confidence

Give yourself positive messages. This will make it much easier to succeed at anything you attempt. Your self-confidence will also be noticed by others, and they may draw personal strength and confidence from it.

Who knows? Together you may accomplish amazing things.

Happiness does not require luxury

Luxurious surroundings are nice, if you can afford them, but they won't make you happy. Think back. Was your happiest birthday dinner the one you ate at a fancy restaurant? Or was it a simpler one you shared with close friends and family gathered around the kitchen table?

Be imperfect, live longer

Our modern culture places so many demands on us that we cannot keep up with them all. There are schedules we have to keep, meetings we have to attend, places we have to go, things we have to buy—it's just too much, and we know it, but we still try to get everything done. We feel we must be perfect in every way, but of course, we can't, and this makes us feel like failures.

By striving for perfection, we damage ourselves both psychologically and physically. Being hard on yourself all the time makes you unhappy, and unhappiness causes your brain to release chemicals that damage your cells. It doesn't have to be that way. You may not be able to answer every email the very second you receive it, but that's okay. Accept the fact that you are imperfect and you'll live a happier, healthier, and longer life.

Passion without limits

If you think you know your passion, then don't hold back. Let it run free. By definition, passion must be without limits. You'll never know what your real passion is until you give it a chance to breathe and grow. If your passion is art, then make sure you find time for it.

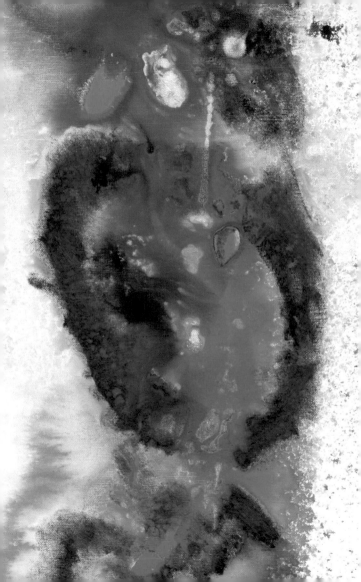

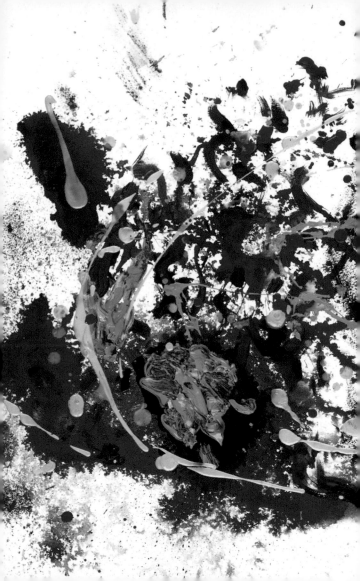

DR. HOWARD MURAD'S INCLUSIVE HEALTH APPROACH

A prominent Los Angeles physician, Dr. Howard Murad has successfully treated more than 50,000 patients. Drawing on his training as both a pharmacist and physician, he has developed a popular and highly effective line of skin care products that has won praise from health- and beauty-conscious people everywhere. A practitioner not just of medicine but of the philosophy of health, he has written dozens of books and articles, earning him a worldwide reputation as an authority on slowing the aging process.

Dr. Murad's approach to medicine is unique. It involves a concept he calls Inclusive Health. An alternative to traditional medical practice with its emphasis on the "spot treatment" of individual conditions or illnesses, the Inclusive Health approach treats the whole patient. Among other things, it considers the patient's diet, lifestyle, and emotional state as well as intercellular water—the hydration level of cells.

Years of painstaking research and experience with thousands of patients have shown Dr. Murad that human health and happiness are directly linked to the ability of cells to retain water. A poor diet and the stress of day-to-day living can damage the all-important membranes that form cell walls. Over time, the membranes become broken and porous, causing the cells to leak water and lose vitality. This, in turn, leads to accelerated aging and a wide variety of diseases and syndromes.

In his groundbreaking bestseller *The Water Secret*, published in 2010, Dr. Murad explained how to stop this process—and reverse it—through Inclusive Healthcare. This approach has three essential components. The first involves good skincare practices; the second, a healthy diet emphasizing raw fruits and vegetables; and the third, an overall reduction in stress combined with a more youthful and creative outlook on life.

The third component, which emphasizes our emotional state, may be the hardest part of the Inclusive Health treatment process for people to adopt. The breakneck pace of modern life with its freeways, computers, cell phones, and fast-paced living creates an enormous amount of what Dr. Murad describes as *cultural stress.*

To deal with this runaway stress, we live increasingly structured lives that are less and less open to the free play and creativity that make life worth living. *We can choose not to live this way.* But reducing stress and embracing a more youthful outlook often involves major shifts in lifestyle—changes in jobs, accommodations, locales, hobbies, habits, and relationships. It may even require a complete personal transformation of the sort sometimes identified with a single galvanizing moment of self-awareness. You may experience a transforming moment like that while walking on a beach, creating a work of art, driving through the countryside, or maybe just stretching your arms after a long night's sleep. Who can say?

To help his patients awaken to a better life, Dr. Murad has composed a substantial collection of personal insights, or

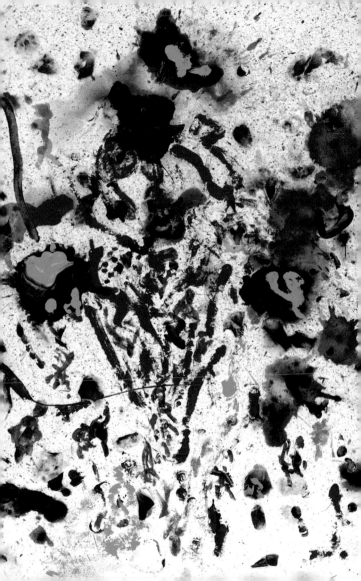

sayings, that deliver bits of health advice, philosophy, and wisdom straight up, like strong coffee. In his medical practice, Dr. Murad shares these brief meditations with patients as a way of encouraging them to improve their health by adopting more youthful, creative, and health-conscious lifestyles. You may find them similarly inspirational. In addition to the insights you have already encountered in this book, here are a few others that you may find interesting and useful.

Encourage your free spirit.

———————

To become younger,
explore your passion.

Transitions are imperfect roadmaps to the future, and it is up to you to make the best of them.

———————————

Become important to yourself.

———————————

Be comfortable with who you are.

———————————

Unlock your hidden potential.

———————————

Don't feel guilty for being yourself.

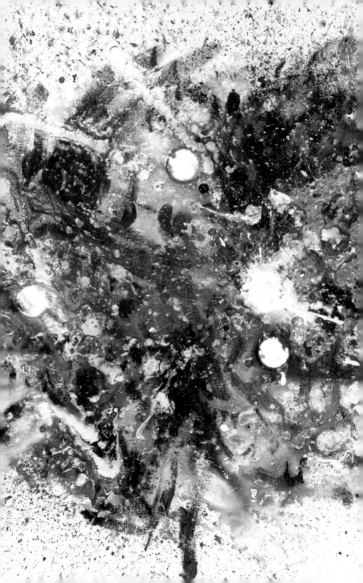

Delete negative self-talk.

Find your hidden potential.

Success comes when you accept the possibility of failure.

If permitted, failure leads to success.

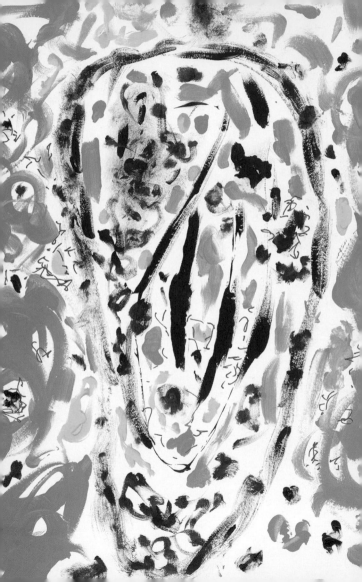

*Take pleasure in every
minor success.*

---

*There is a difference between
having fun and being happy.*

---

*Give yourself permission to
make your own journey.*

---

*Give yourself permission to
have your own opinion.*

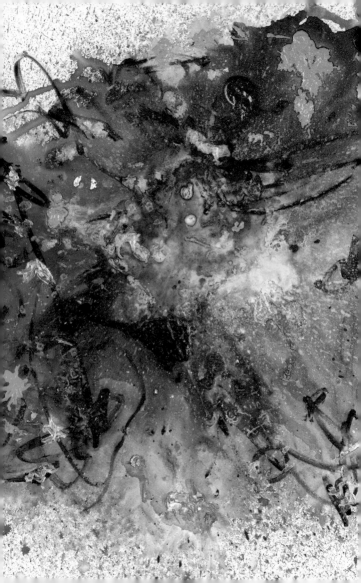

Don't feel guilty for being yourself.

Don't blame yourself for other people's problems.

Medicine is imperfect; you have to look at it inclusively.

We are each born with a unique commodity called life. It is stressed by the environment, and it is up to us to make the best of it.

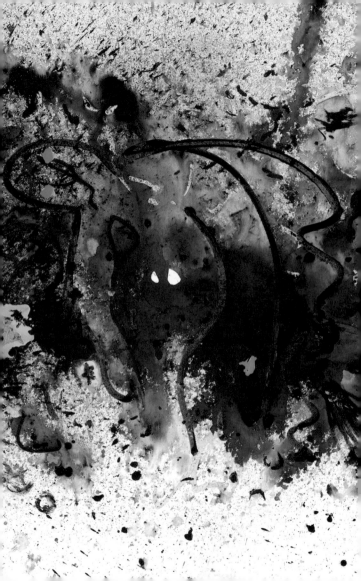

Dear reader,
Please share this book with others or give it as a gift to family, friends, or business associates. Also, be sure to look for Dr. Murad's other inspirational "little" books:

*Why Have a Bad Day
When You Can Have a Good Day?*

Be Imperfect—Live Longer

One Key Can Open Many Doors

Honor Yourself

The Best Is Yet to Come

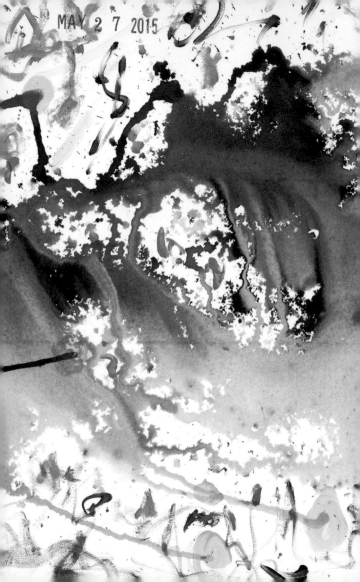

MAY 2 7 2015